THE *Skinny*
TAKEAWAY
RECIPE BOOK

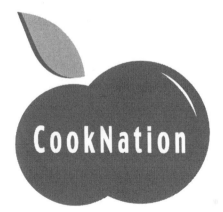

CookNation

The Skinny Takeaway Recipe Book
Healthier Versions Of Your Fast Food Favourites: Chinese, Indian, Pizza, Burgers, Southern Style Chicken, Mexican & More. All Under 300, 400 & 500 Calories.

Copyright
Copyright © Bell & Mackenzie Publishing Limited 2014

ISBN 978-1-909855-55-7

A CIP catalogue record of this book is available from the British Library

Disclaimer
Some recipes may contain nuts or traces of nuts. Those suffering from any allergies associated with nuts should avoid any recipes containing nuts or nut based oils.
This information is provided and sold with the knowledge that the publisher and author do not offer any legal or other professional advice.
In the case of a need for any such expertise consult with the appropriate professional.
This book does not contain all information available on the subject, and other sources of recipes are available.
This book has not been created to be specific to any individual's requirements.
Every effort has been made to make this book as accurate as possible. However, there may be typographical and or content errors. Therefore, this book should serve only as a general guide and not as the ultimate source of subject information.
This book contains information that might be dated and is intended only to educate and entertain.
The author and publisher shall have no liability or responsibility to any person or entity regarding any loss or damage incurred, or alleged to have incurred, directly or indirectly, by the information contained in this book.

Contents

Contents

Contents

Contents

INTRODUCTION

If we are all completely honest with ourselves, takeaway food tastes great!
Nothing else quite hits the spot. We all crave some kind of fast food takeaway on a regular basis whether it's Chinese on a Friday night, fish & chips for dinner, pizza after the cinema or a curry with friends. Our fast-paced busy lives, convenience food outlets everywhere you turn and relentless advertising make the opportunity to consume more and more takeaway fast food hard to resist!

The significance however of consuming too much unhealthy food is a cause for concern. Takeaway food whilst tasting good, instant and satisfying is more often than not packed with additional calories with excessive fat, sugar and salt which can all be contributing factors to serious health problems such as heart disease, diabetes, high cholesterol and obesity.

Moreover if you are following a calorie controlled diet, one moment of takeaway weakness, can throw your hard earned weight loss efforts to the wind in one fell swoop. When was the last time you saw calories listed on a Chinese takeaway menu?!

But takeaway food tastes so good!
Yes it does and rewarding yourself with your favourite fast food every now again isn't really such a bad thing. But what if you could eat some of your favourite takeaway treats more often without feeling guilty, without destroying your diet or weight management program, without consuming more than the recommended levels of fat, sugar and salt and without noticing a hole in your purse?

How?
By making your own healthier, simpler, lower fat, lower calorie.....skinnier versions of your favourite takeaway and fast foods at home. Takeaway temptation can be satisfied by making just a few simple and choice swaps in the ingredients that are lower in fat and calories without compromising on taste. For example; for Pizza we suggest thin crust bases with lean toppings and tomato-based sauces avoiding deep stuffed crusts and excessive cheese. If you like oriental food, steamed dumplings & stir-fry's are better options than battered prawn balls with a thick sugary sauce. Maybe you love chips: bigger, thicker chips will absorb less fat then small 'French fries' but why not try baked sweet potato fries as an alternative? Delicious!

With *The Skinny Takeaway Recipe Book* you can choose from over 70 versions of delicious fast food meals, dishes, sides & snacks served at many of the most popular takeaway and fast food outlets.

Our recipes include skinny, healthier versions of some of the best-loved takeaway treats in the UK. All recipes are simple, most can be prepared and cooked in under 30 minutes, are cheaper than the takeaway version, but most importantly….they are skinnier - meaning you can still enjoy a version of your favoured takeaway treat guilt-free!

Choose your takeaway/fast food dish from:

Chinese **Kebabs** **Mexican** **Thai**
Pizza **Burgers**
Indian **Southen Style Chicken**

The Skinny Takeaway Fast Food Recipe Book doesn't glorify the consumption of fast food or justify or encourage the concept of modern mass produced meals. Nor does it claim to reveal the hidden secrets of takeaway restaurants around the country. Our recipes, whilst delicious and healthier don't claim to taste exactly like the ones you might usually order for takeaway. If the truth be told, you are unlikely to replicate the taste of Kentucky Fried Chicken at home without a whole lot of fat for deep-frying and a good helping of Monosodium Glutamate (MSG).

Here are the ingredients for KFC Hot Wings as listed on their website at ***www.kfc.com/nutrition***
Breaded Chicken Wing Sections, Salt, Seasoning (Monosodium Glutamate, Spice, Extractives of Spice, Garlic Powder) and Sodium Phosphates. Battered With: Water, Bleached Wheat Flour, Modified Corn Starch, Seasoning (Monosodium Glutamate, Spice, Extractives of Spice and Garlic Powder), Yellow Corn Flour, Salt. Breaded With: Bleached Wheat Flour. Predusted With: Bleached Wheat Flour, Modified Corn Starch, Yellow Corn Flour, Salt. Breading Set in Vegetable Oil.

Compare this to the ingredients for our **Skinny Hot Wings**
12 skinless chicken wings, 250ml/1 cup low fat buttermilk, 2 tbsp plain flour,1 tsp each ground black pepper, cayenne pepper & garlic powder, ½ tsp salt, 20g/1oz low fat 'butter' spread, 3 tbsp fat free Greek yoghurt, 2 tbsp freshly chopped chives, salt & pepper to taste.

Notice the difference?

Our recipes offer healthier alternatives to your favourite takeaway and fast food treats that are lower in calories, fat & sugar than those you would ordinarily order on your local high street.

Resisting the temptation to order in your usual takeaway does of course take a little willpower but thinking ahead and planning your meals means you can have your store-cupboard stocked with everything you need to make your takeaway treat at home any day of the week. In most cases, preparation and cooking times will be less than the time you would have to wait for your regular order to be delivered or to collect.

Most independent takeaway restaurants do not display calorie counts for their meals although some of the larger established chains now do, albeit in very small print! Making a healthier choice when ordering takeaway can be impossible.

Did you know that a Chicken korma with pilau rice can stack up to **1000 calories** before you even add naan bread or poppadums while a sweet and sour pork with special fried rice can be a whopping **1100 calories**! The pattern is similar when you look at the most popular fast food choices. It's easy to see why, if we are not careful, that takeaway fast foods can lead to bad health choices and weight gain.

With each of our skinny recipes we offer healthier ingredients that slash the calorie count and introduce you to alternative ways of preparing your chosen dish.

If you enjoy takeaway and fast food treats as much as we do you'll love our skinny recipes, and with The Skinny Takeaway Recipe Book we think you'll agree *Diet can still mean Delicious!*

About CookNation

CookNation is the leading publisher of innovative and practical recipe books for the modern, health-conscious cook.

CookNation titles bring together delicious, easy and practical recipes with their unique approach - easy and delicious, no-nonsense recipes - making cooking for diets and healthy eating fast, simple and fun.

With a range of #1 best-selling titles - from the innovative 'Skinny' calorie-counted series, to the 5:2 Diet Recipes collection - CookNation recipe books prove that 'Diet' can still mean 'Delicious'!

Turn to the end of this book to browse all CookNation's recipe books

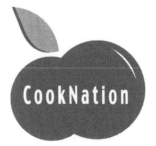

Skinny
CHINESE
&THAI

Hong Kong Style Sweet & Sour Chicken

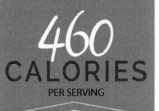

460 CALORIES PER SERVING

Ingredients   Serves 4

500g/1lb 2oz skinless, chicken breast
1 red pepper, deseeded & sliced
½ onion, sliced
400g/14oz tinned pineapple chunks,
reserve the juice
2 tsp tamarind paste
1 tbsp brown sugar
60ml/¼ cup rice wine vinegar

200g/7oz rice
Low cal cooking oil spray
Salt & pepper to taste

Chefs Note
Make sure you taste the sauce whilst it's cooking as you may need to balance the sugar and vinegar a little to get it just right.

1. Preheat the oven to 400f/200c/Gas 6

2. Season the chicken and spray with a little low cal oil. Cover with foil and cook in a preheated oven for 30 minutes or until cooked through.

3. Place the sliced peppers, onions & reserved pineapple juice in a blender and blend until pureed. Add the puree to a saucepan & quickly bring to the boil.

4. Reduce the heat to a gentle simmer and add the pineapple chunks, tamarind paste, sugar and vinegar. Cover and leave to simmer whilst the chicken cooks.

5. Meanwhile cook the rice in salted boiling water until tender.

6. When the chicken is cooked cut into cubes, add to the saucepan and combine well.

7. Serve the drained rice with the sweet & sour chicken piled on top.

Chicken Chow Mein

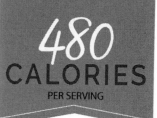

480 CALORIES PER SERVING

Ingredients Serves 4

1 tbsp fresh grated ginger
4 tbsp oyster sauce
4 tbsp soy sauce
2 garlic cloves, crushed
60ml/¼ cup ketchup
1 tbsp vegetable oil
300g/11oz skinless, chicken breast, thinly sliced

1 red pepper, deseeded & sliced
1 onion, sliced
250g/9oz dried noodles
1 chicken stock cube
200g/7oz fresh beansprouts
Salt & pepper to taste

1. Mix together the ginger, oyster sauce, soy sauce, garlic & ketchup to make a sauce.

2. Season the chicken and heat the oil in a wok or large frying pan.

3. Quickly brown the chicken for a minute or two along with the sliced peppers & onions. Add the sauce and continue to cook for 2-3 minutes.

4. Meanwhile cook the noodles in boiling water, along with the chicken stock cube, until tender.

5. Drain the noodles and quickly add to the wok along with the beansprouts.

6. Toss everything really well. Check the chicken is cooked through, season & serve.

Chefs Note

Finely sliced spring onions make a great garnish to this popular takeaway dish.

Egg Fried Rice

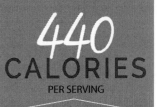

Ingredients   Serves 4

400g/14oz rice (reduce by half if using as a side dish)
1 vegetable or chicken stock cube, crumbled
1 tbsp vegetable oil
2 free range eggs, use the whites only

1 tsp sesame oil
2 tbsp soy sauce
125g/4oz peas
Salt & pepper to taste

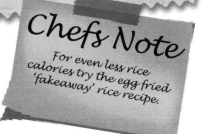

Chefs Note
For even less rice calories try the egg fried 'fakeaway' rice recipe.

1. First cook the rice in salted boiling water, along with the crumbled stock cube, until tender. Drain and leave to cool completely (or use precooked rice if you wish).

2. Beat together the egg whites, sesame oil & soy sauce.

3. Cook the peas and put to one side.

4. Heat the vegetable oil in a wok or large frying pan. Add the cooled rice and stir-fry on a high heat for 2-3 minutes. Make sure the rice is separated and not stuck together.

5. Make a well in the centre of the rice and pour in the egg white mixture. Allow it to set for about 10-15 seconds and then quickly beat the setting egg strands through the rice.

6. Keep the rice moving, add the peas and make sure everything is piping hot before seasoning and serving.

Fakeaway Egg Fried Rice

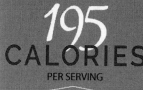

195 CALORIES PER SERVING

Ingredients Serves 4

2 cauliflower heads (just use one if using as a side dish)
1 garlic clove, peeled
1 tbsp vegetable oil
2 free range eggs, use the whites only
1 tsp sesame oil

2 tbsp soy sauce
125g/4oz peas
Salt & pepper to taste

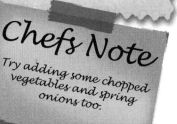

Chefs Note
Try adding some chopped vegetables and spring onions too.

1. Place the cauliflower and garlic in a food processor and pulse until the cauliflower turns into rice sized grains.

2. Place the 'rice' in a microwavable dish and cook covered for 4-5 minutes or until the 'rice' is piping hot.

3. Meanwhile mix together the egg whites, sesame oil & soy sauce and cook the peas.

4. Heat the vegetable oil in a wok or large frying pan. Add the 'rice' and stir-fry for a minute.

5. Make a well in the centre of the rice and pour in the egg white mixture. Allow it to set for about 10-15 seconds and then quickly beat the setting egg strands through the rice.

6. Keep the rice moving, add the peas and make sure everything is piping hot before seasoning and serving.

Singapore Noodles

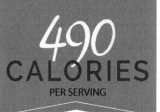
Ingredients   Serves 4

1 tbsp curry powder
6 tbsp soy sauce
2 tbsp rice wine vinegar
1 tsp brown sugar
3 garlic cloves, crushed
120ml/½ cup chicken stock
1 tbsp vegetable oil
150g/5oz shelled king prawns, chopped

150g/5oz chicken breast, finely sliced
125g/4oz frozen peas, defrosted
½ onion, sliced
½ pointed cabbage, finely shredded
300g/11oz dried vermicelli noodles
1 chicken stock cube, crumbled
2 free range eggs, whites only
Salt & pepper to taste

Chefs Note
Use medium or hot curry powder depending on your preference.

1. Mix together the curry powder, soy sauce, vinegar, brown sugar, garlic & stock to make a sauce

2. Season the chicken & prawns and heat the vegetable oil in a wok or large frying pan. Add to the pan and quickly brown the chicken and pink-up the prawns for a minute or two along with the peas, onions & shredded cabbage. Add the sauce and continue to stir-fry for 2-3 minutes on a high heat.

3. Meanwhile cook the noodles in boiling water, along with the crumbled chicken stock cube, until tender.

4. Drain the noodles and quickly add to the wok along with the eggs whites.

5. Toss everything really well. Check the chicken and prawns are cooked through and the egg whites have set into strands. Season & serve.

Lemon Chicken

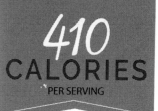

410 CALORIES PER SERVING

Ingredients   Serves 4

500g/1lb 2oz skinless, chicken breast
1 tbsp cornflour
6 tbsp lemon juice
1 tbsp runny honey
2 tbsp soy sauce
250ml/1 cup chicken stock

1 carrot, peeled & sliced into matchsticks
1 red pepper, deseeded & finely sliced
½ onion, sliced
200g/7oz rice
Low cal cooking oil spray
Salt & pepper to taste

1. Preheat the oven to 400f/200c/Gas 6

2. Season the chicken and spray with a little low cal oil. Cover with foil and cook in a preheated oven for 30 minutes or until cooked through.

Chefs Note

The sauce should be sticky and sweet with the cornflour helping to thicken the finished dish.

3. Meanwhile mix the cornflour with a little warm water to make a paste.

4. Place the lemon juice, honey, soy sauce & stock in a saucepan and bring to the boil. Reduce the heat and gently stir through the cornflour paste.

5. Add the carrots, peppers & onions to the saucepan, cover and leave to gently simmer whilst the chicken cooks.

6. Whilst the sauce is simmering cook the rice in salted boiling water until tender.

7. When the chicken is cooked quickly cut into cubes. Add to saucepan and combine well.

8. Serve the drained rice with the lemon chicken piled on top.

Kung Pao Chicken

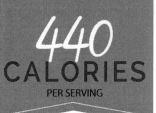

Ingredients   Serves 4

500g/1lb 2oz skinless, chicken breast, cubed
2 tsp cornflour
1 tbsp balsamic vinegar
1 tbsp hoisin sauce
2 tbsp soy sauce
1 tsp crushed dried chillies
2 garlic cloves, crushes

200g/7oz rice
1 tbsp vegetable oil
1 large bunch spring onions, sliced lengthways
Salt & pepper to taste

Chefs Note

To coat the chicken, place the chicken in a plastic bag with the flour and shake well until evenly covered.

1. Season the chicken and coat with the cornflour.

2. Mix together the balsamic vinegar, hoisin sauce, soy sauce, chillies & garlic together to make a sauce.

3. Cook the rice in salted boiling water until tender.

4. Meanwhile heat the oil in a wok or large frying pan. Add the chicken and brown for 2-3 minutes. Add the sauce and continue to cook until the chicken is cooked through and sticky (add a splash of water to the pan if needed).

5. Serve the drained rice with the sticky chicken and the sliced spring onions sprinkled over the top

Salt & Pepper Prawns

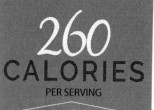

260 CALORIES PER SERVING

Ingredients   Serves 4

1 tbsp ground black peppercorns
1 tsp Chinese five spice powder
1 tbsp crushed sea salt flakes
500g/1lb 2oz shelled raw king prawns
2 tbsp vegetable oil
3 garlic cloves, finely sliced
2 red chillies, deseeded & finely sliced

1 large bunch spring onions, sliced
Salt & pepper to taste

1. Mix together the ground black pepper, five spice powder & sea salt. Add to a plastic bag and toss the prawns in. Shake well until the prawns are evenly covered.

2. Meanwhile heat the oil in a wok or large frying pan. Add the sliced garlic, chillies, spring onions & prawns and stir-fry for 3-5 minutes or until the prawns are cooked through.

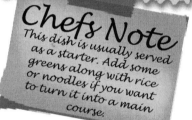

Chefs Note
This dish is usually served as a starter. Add some greens along with rice or noodles if you want to turn it into a main course.

Chicken & Sweetcorn Soup

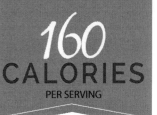

160 CALORIES PER SERVING

Ingredients   Serves 4

250g/9oz skinless, chicken breast
2 tsp freshly grated ginger
2 garlic cloves, crushed
1.25lt/5 cups chicken stock

250g/9oz sweetcorn
2 free range eggs, whites only
Low cal cooking oil spray
Salt & pepper to taste

Chefs Note
Serve with a dash of soy sauce and a little fresh, chopped chilli if you like.

1. Preheat the oven to 400f/200c/Gas 6

2. Season the chicken and spray with a little low cal oil. Cover with foil and cook in a preheated oven for 30 minutes or until cooked through.

3. When the chicken is cooked shred as finely as possible with two forks.

4. Add the shredded chicken, ginger, garlic, stock & sweetcorn to a saucepan. Bring to the boil and leave to simmer for 3-5 minutes or until everything is cooked through and piping hot.

5. Beat the egg whites in a cup and swirl through the soup until they begin to set into egg strands.

6. Remove from the heat. Season and serve.

Beef & Peppers In Black Bean Sauce

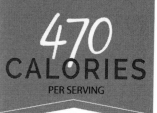

470 CALORIES PER SERVING

Ingredients
Serves 4

200g/7oz rice
500g/1lb 2oz good quality lean steak
2 green peppers, deseeded & cut into chunks
1 onion, sliced
2 garlic cloves, crushed
6 tbsp black bean sauce
150g/5oz fresh beansprouts

Low cal cooking oil spray
Salt & pepper to taste

1. Cook the rice in salted boiling water until tender.

2. Meanwhile trim any fat off the steak, season and thinly slice.

Chefs Note
Black bean sauce is made from fermented, salt-preserved soya beans so it's not realistic to expect to make it from scratch. Jar bought is fine!

3. Spray a little low cal oil in a frying pan or wok and gently stir fry the peppers, onions and garlic for a few minutes until softened. Add a dash of water if the pan needs loosening up a little.

4. Increase the heat and add the sliced steak, black bean sauce & beansprouts. Stir-fry for 2-4 minutes or until the steak is cooked to your liking.

5. Serve the drained rice with the steak piled on top.

Beef & Broccoli In Oyster Sauce

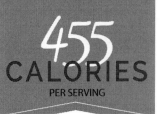

455 CALORIES PER SERVING

Ingredients   Serves 4

200g/7oz rice
500g/1lb 2oz good quality lean steak
2 tsp cornflour
½ tsp Chinese five spice powder
1 red pepper, deseeded & cut into chunks
200g/7oz tenderstem broccoli roughly chopped
1 onion, sliced

½ tsp crushed dried chilli flakes
2 tbsp rice wine vinegar
3 tbsp soy sauce
120ml/½ cup chicken stock
3 tbsp oyster sauce
Low cal cooking oil spray
Salt & pepper to taste

Chefs Note
Blanch the broccoli first if you prefer it more tender.

1. Cook the rice in salted boiling water until tender.

2. Meanwhile trim any fat off the steak. Give it a good bash with a meat hammer, season and thinly slice.

3. Mix the beef strips with the cornflour and Chinese five spice powder until even covered.

4. Spray a little low cal oil in a frying pan or wok and gently stir-fry the peppers, broccoli and onions for a few minutes until softened. Add a dash of water if the pan needs loosening up a little.

5. Increase the heat and add the sliced steak. Cook for 2 minutes before adding the chilli flakes, rice wine vinegar, soy sauce, chicken stock and oyster sauce.

6. Continue stir-frying until the sauce thickens up and the dish is piping hot.

7. Serve the drained rice with the steak piled on top.

Ginger, Beef & Pineapple

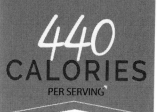

Ingredients   Serves 4

200g/7oz rice
500g/1lb 2oz good quality lean steak
1 red chilli, deseeded & finely chopped
1 tbsp rice wine vinegar
2 tsp brown sugar
3 tbsp soy sauce

1 onion, sliced
1 tbsp freshly grated ginger
300g/11oz tinned pineapple chunks, drained
Low cal cooking oil spray
Salt & pepper to taste

1. Trim any fat off the steak, season and thinly slice. Place in a bowl with the chopped chilli, vinegar, brown sugar & soy sauce. Combine well and leave to marinade for 15-20 minutes.

2. Cook the rice in salted boiling water until tender.

3. Meanwhile spray a little low cal oil in a frying pan or wok and gently stir-fry the onions & ginger for a few minutes until softened. Add a dash of water if the pan needs loosening up a little.

4. Increase the heat and add the marinated steak & pineapples chunks. Stir-fry until the sauce thickens up and the dish is piping hot.

5. Serve with the drained rice.

Chefs Note

If you are short of time 'lazy' pre-chopped ginger will work well.

Prawn Dim Sum

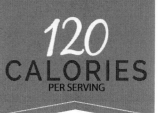

120 CALORIES PER SERVING

Ingredients   Serves 4

2 tbsp soy sauce
½ tsp each salt & brown sugar
250g/9oz raw king prawns
1 spring onion

2 tsp grated ginger
16 pre-made dim sum cases
Bamboo steamer

Chefs Note

Bamboo steamers are very cheap to buy and simple to use. Dim sum wrappers are widely available in Asian supermarkets.

1. Mix the soy sauce, salt & sugar together until the sugar and salt dissolves.

2. Place this soy mixture, along with the prawns, spring onions & grated ginger, in a food processor and pulse until finely minced.

3. Lay out the dim sum wrappers and divide the prawn mixture evenly between the cases: placing the minced prawn into the centre of each flat case, fold over to create a semi circle and seal by squeezing the edges together.

4. Place the dumplings in a bamboo steamer and steam for 5-7 minutes or until cooked through and piping hot.

5. Serve with soy sauce.

Stir-Fried Chinese Mushrooms

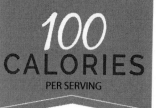

100
CALORIES
PER SERVING

Ingredients   Serves 4

2 tsp sesame oil
3 garlic cloves, crushed
2 tsp grated fresh ginger
400g/14oz Chinese
shitake mushrooms, sliced

2 tbsp soy sauce
1 bunch spring onions, sliced
Salt & pepper to taste

1. Add the sesame oil to a frying pan or wok and gently stir fry the garlic and ginger for 2 minutes.

2. Increase the heat, add the mushrooms, soy sauce & spring onions and cook until the mushrooms are soft and cooked through. Add a dash of water if the pan needs loosening up a little.

3. Season and serve.

Chefs Note

This is usually served as a side dish. You could serve with rice or noodles if you wanted to make it a main course.

Prawn Pad Thai

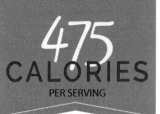

475 CALORIES PER SERVING

Ingredients   Serves 4

3 tbsp lime juice
1 tsp each cayenne pepper, brown sugar & grated ginger
4 tbsp fish sauce
4 tbsp soy sauce
2 garlic cloves, crushed
1 tbsp vegetable oil
300g/11oz raw, shelled king prawns

300g/11oz dried noodles
1 chicken stock cube
200g/7oz fresh beansprouts
25g/1oz chopped peanuts
Salt & pepper to taste

Chefs Note

Thick udon noodles are ideal for Pad Thai.

1. Mix together the lime juice, cayenne pepper, brown sugar, ginger, fish sauce, soy sauce & crushed garlic to make a sauce.

2. Season the prawns and heat the oil in a wok or large frying pan. Quickly saute the prawns for a minute or two. Add the sauce and continue to cook for 2-3 minutes.

3. Meanwhile cook the noodles in boiling water, along with the crumbled chicken stock cube, until tender.

4. Drain the noodles and quickly add to the wok along with the beansprouts.

5. Toss everything really well, cook for a further 2 minutes. Season & serve with the chopped peanuts on top.

Chicken Thai Green Curry

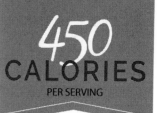

450 CALORIES PER SERVING

Ingredients   Serves 4

500g/1lb 2oz skinless, chicken breast
1 onion, sliced
1 garlic clove, crushed
200g/7oz green beans, roughly chopped
2 tbsp Thai green curry paste
2 tsp fish sauce
120ml/½ cup low fat coconut milk

200g/7oz rice
Low cal cooking oil spray
Salt & pepper to taste

1. Cut the chicken into slices & season,

2. Gently saute the onion, garlic & green beans in a little low cal spray for a few minutes until softened (loosen the pan with a splash of water if needed).

Chefs Note

This curry is great served with lime wedges.

3. Add the chicken, curry paste, fish sauce & coconut milk. Combine well, cover and leave on a very gentle simmer for 10-12 minutes.

4. Meanwhile cook the rice in salted boiling water until tender.

5. When the chicken is cooked through. Serve the drained rice with the Thai chicken curry piled on top.

Chilli Beef Ramen

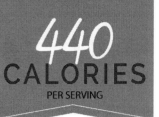

440 CALORIES PER SERVING

Ingredients   Serves 4

2 tsp paprika
300g/11oz lean sirloin steak
1.25lt/5 cups chicken stock
2 garlic cloves, crushed
1 tbsp freshly grated ginger
2 red chillies, deseeded & finely chopped

300g/11oz dried ramen noodles
2 pak choi, shredded
1 large bunch spring onions, sliced
Salt & pepper to taste

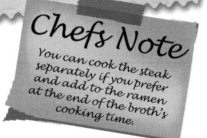

Chefs Note

You can cook the steak separately if you prefer and add to the ramen at the end of the broth's cooking time.

1. Brush the steak with the paprika and slice up into the thinnest slivers you can manage.

2. Place the stock in a saucepan on a high heat until it is simmering. Add the garlic, ginger & chillies and leave to cook for 2 minutes. Add the ramen noodles & shredded pak choi and continue simmering for a further 2-3 minutes or until the noodles are tender.

3. Toss in the steak & chopped spring onions and cook for just one minute in the boiling broth until the steak is just cooked and the spring onions are still crunchy.

4. Divide into bowls and serve straight away.

Skinny
CURRY

Chicken Korma

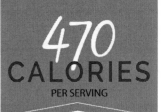

470 CALORIES PER SERVING

Ingredients   Serves 4

3 garlic cloves, crushed
2 carrots, chopped
1 onion, sliced
2 bay leaves
400g/14oz tinned chopped tomatoes
2 tbsp tomato puree
120ml/½ cup chicken stock
1 tsp each brown sugar & salt

2 tbsp mild curry powder
500g/1lb 2oz skinless, chicken breast cubed
1 tbsp coconut cream
20g/1oz ground almonds
200g/7oz rice
Low cal cooking oil spray
Salt & pepper

Chefs Note
Ground almonds give this Korma its distinctive texture.

1. Gently sautee the garlic, carrots & onions in a little low cal spray for a few minutes until softened. Add the bay leaves, chopped tomatoes, puree, stock, sugar, salt & curry powder. Stir well, cover and leave to gently simmer for 30 minutes.

2. After this time remove the bay leaves and discard. Place the sauce in a blender and blend until smooth. Return to the pan, add the chicken and cook for 20 minutes or cooked through.

3. Meanwhile cook the rice in salted boiling water until tender.

4. Stir the coconut cream and ground almonds through the curry and serve piled on top of the drained rice.

Lamb Vindaloo

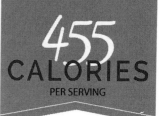

Ingredients   Serves 4

3 garlic cloves, crushed
2 carrots, chopped
400g/14oz tinned chopped tomatoes
2 tbsp tomato puree
120ml/½ cup chicken stock
1 tsp each brown sugar & salt

1 tsp each chilli powder, cayenne pepper, coriander, cumin, turmeric & garam masala
1 onion, sliced
500g/1lb 2oz lean lamb fillet, cubed
200g/7oz rice
Low cal cooking oil spray
Salt & pepper to taste

1. Gently saute the garlic & carrots in a little low cal spray for a few minutes until softened. Add the chopped tomatoes, puree, stock, sugar, salt & dried spices. Stir well, cover and leave to gently simmer for 30 minutes.

Chefs Note

You may like to serve with a cooling yoghurt dip on the side!

2. After this time remove to a blender and blend to make a smooth sauce. Return to the pan and add the sliced onions. Quickly brown the lamb in a hot pan with a little low cal spray for a minute or two until the meat is sealed. Add the lamb to the sauce, cover and simmer for 20-30 minutes or until the lamb is cooked through.

3. Meanwhile cook the rice in salted boiling water until tender.

4. Check the seasoning & 'heat' of the curry and serve piled on top of the drained rice.

Chicken Bhuna

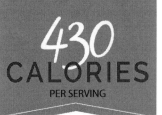

Ingredients   Serves 4

2 garlic cloves, crushed
1 onion, chopped
400g/14oz tinned chopped tomatoes
2 tbsp tomato puree
120ml/½ cup chicken stock
1 tsp each brown sugar, salt, ground turmeric, chilli powder, fenugreek seeds, ginger, coriander, cumin & garam masala

500g/1lb 2oz skinless, chicken breast cubed
2 carrots, cut into batons
150g/4oz peas
1 red pepper deseeded & sliced
2 tbsp fat free Greek yoghurt
1 tbsp lemon juice
200g/7oz rice
Low cal cooking oil spray
Salt & pepper

Chefs Note
Use whichever mix of vegetables you have to hand for this recipe in place of carrots, peas & peppers.

1. Gently saute the garlic & onions in a little low cal spray for a few minutes until softened. Add the chopped tomatoes, puree, stock, sugar, salt & dried spices. Stir well, cover and leave to gently simmer for 30 minutes.

2. After this time remove to a blender and blend to make a smooth sauce. Return to the pan, add the chicken, carrots, peas & peppers and cook for 20 minutes or until the chicken is cooked through and the carrots are tender.

3. Meanwhile cook the rice in salted boiling water until tender.

4. Stir the yoghurt & lemon juice through the curry and serve on top of the drained rice.

Rogan Josh

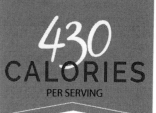

430 CALORIES PER SERVING

Ingredients
Serves 4

3 garlic cloves, crushed
1 onion, chopped
1 carrot, chopped
400g/14oz tinned chopped tomatoes
2 tbsp tomato puree
120ml/½ cup chicken stock
1 tsp each brown sugar & salt
1 tbsp medium curry powder
1 tsp each turmeric & paprika
½ tsp each ground cinnamon & cloves
500g/1lb 2oz skinless, chicken breast cubed
200g/7oz fresh tomatoes, roughly chopped
200g/7oz rice
Low cal cooking oil spray
Salt & pepper to taste

1. Gently saute the garlic, onions & carrots in a little low cal spray for a few minutes until softened. Add the tinned tomatoes, puree, stock, sugar, salt, curry powder & dried spices. Stir well, cover and leave to gently simmer for 30 minutes.

Chefs Note

Rogan josh should be an aromatic curry but you can reduce the cinnamon & cloves if you prefer.

2. After this time remove to a blender and blend to make a smooth sauce. Return to the pan, add the chicken & fresh tomatoes and cook for 20 minutes or until the chicken is cooked through.

3. Meanwhile cook the rice in salted boiling water until tender.

4. Check the seasoning of the curry and serve piled on top of the drained rice.

Chicken Jalfrezi

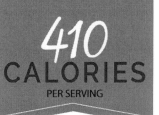

410 CALORIES
PER SERVING

Ingredients   Serves 4

3 garlic cloves, crushed
2 carrots, chopped
400g/14oz tinned chopped tomatoes
2 tbsp tomato puree
120ml/½ cup chicken stock
1 tsp each brown sugar & salt
1 tsp each ground ginger, coriander, cumin, turmeric & garam masala
½ tsp chilli powder
500g/1lb 2oz skinless, chicken breast cubed
3 green chillies, deseeded & finely sliced
2 onions, sliced
200g/7oz rice
Low cal cooking oil spray
Salt & pepper to taste

Chefs Note
Fresh chillies are synonymous with Jalfrezi. Feel free to adjust to suit your own taste

1. Gently saute the garlic & carrots in a little low cal spray for a few minutes until softened. Add the chopped tomatoes, puree, stock, sugar, salt & dried spices. Stir well, cover and leave to gently simmer for 30 minutes.

2. After this time remove to a blender and blend to make a smooth sauce. Return to the pan, add the chicken, chillies & sliced onions and cook for 20 minutes or until the chicken is cooked through.

3. Meanwhile cook the rice in salted boiling water until tender.

4. Check the seasoning of the curry and serve piled on top of the drained rice.

Tikka Masala

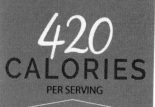
Ingredients Serves 4

500g/1lb 2oz skinless, chicken breast cubed
1 tsp each ground coriander, turmeric, cumin & garam masala
1 tbsp lemon juice
3 garlic cloves, crushed
2 carrots, chopped
1 onion, sliced

400g/14oz tinned chopped tomatoes
2 tbsp tomato puree
120ml/½ cup chicken stock
1 tsp each brown sugar & salt
1 tbsp medium curry powder
4 tbsp fat free Greek Yoghurt
200g/7oz rice
Low cal cooking oil spray
Salt & pepper to taste

1. Mix together the chicken, coriander, turmeric, cumin, garam masala & lemon juice until the chicken is completely covered with the spices. Cover and leave to marinade.

Chefs Note
Leave the chicken to marinate overnight if possible.

2. Gently saute the garlic, carrots & sliced onions in a little low cal spray for a few minutes until softened. Add the chopped tomatoes, puree, stock, sugar, salt & curry powder. Stir well, cover and leave to gently simmer for 30 minutes.

3. Meanwhile preheat the oven grill. Spray the marinated chicken pieces with low cal oil and cook under a medium heat for 6-12 minutes or until cooked through.

4. Cook the rice in salted boiling water until tender.

5. After the saucepan, containing chopped tomatoes, has simmered for 30 minutes remove to a blender and blend to make a smooth sauce. Return to the pan, add the cooked chicken & yoghurt. Stir through and serve piled on top of the drained rice.

Garlic Chilli Chicken

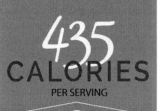

435 CALORIES PER SERVING

Ingredients Serves 4

2 carrots, chopped
1 onion, chopped
400g/14oz tinned chopped tomatoes
2 tbsp tomato puree
120ml/½ cup chicken stock
1 tsp each brown sugar & salt
1 tsp each ground turmeric, paprika, coriander & cumin

500g/1lb 2oz skinless, chicken breast cubed
8 garlic cloves, peeled & thinly sliced
2 green chillies, deseeded & finely sliced
2 large beef tomatoes, roughly chopped
200g/7oz rice
Low cal cooking oil spray
Salt & pepper

Chefs Note
Naturally this dish is heavy on garlic & chilli. Adjust to suit your own palate.

1. Gently saute the carrots & onions in a little low cal spray for a few minutes until softened. Add the tinned tomatoes, puree, stock, sugar, salt & dried spices. Stir well, cover and leave to gently simmer for 30 minutes.

2. After this time remove to a blender, blend to make a smooth sauce and return to the pan.

3. Gently saute the chicken breast, sliced garlic & chillies in a frying pan with a little low cal spray for a minute or two until the meat is sealed and the garlic begins to soften (loosen the pan with a splash of water if needed). Add these to the sauce and cook for 20 minutes or until the chicken is cooked through.

4. Meanwhile cook the rice in salted boiling water until tender.

5. Check the seasoning and serve the curry on top of the drained rice.

Skinny
PIZZA

Thin Crust Pizza Base

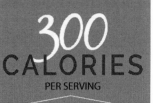
Ingredients   Makes 2 Thin Bases

2.5g/¾ tsp dried yeast
165g/5½oz strong white bread flour
Pinch of salt

Pinch of caster sugar
120ml/½ cup warm water

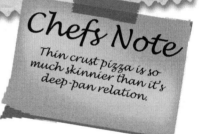

Chefs Note
Thin crust pizza is so much skinnier than it's deep-pan relation.

1. Combine all the ingredients together by hand or use a mixer. Work the ingredients until the dough comes together to form a ball. Use your hands to knead the dough well on a floured surface for about 8 minutes until it becomes soft and springy. Place the dough in a bowl, cover with cling film and leave to rest at room temperature for 15 minutes. After this time split the dough in half and roll out into two thin bases. The thinner the better.

2. Choose your toppings, cover the bases with these and cook in a preheated oven at 220C/450F/Gas Mark 8 for 8-12 minutes or until cooked through and piping hot.

Pepperoni Pizza

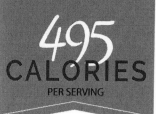

Ingredients   Makes 2 Pizzas

2 homemade pizza bases (see page 38 for recipe)

200g/7oz ripe plum tomatoes, chopped

1 tbsp dried basil

2 garlic cloves, crushed

6 tbsp tomato puree/paste

100g/3 ½oz grated low fat mozzarella cheese

50g/2oz lean pepperoni slices, chopped

Salt & pepper to taste

1. Preheat the oven to 220C/450F/Gas Mark 8 and roll out the pizza bases.

2. Mix together the chopped tomatoes, basil & garlic. Spread the tomato puree evenly over the two bases. Add the chopped tomatoes mix along with the grated cheese and the chopped pepperoni slices.

3. Place in the oven and cook for 8-12 minutes or until golden brown, cooked through and piping hot.

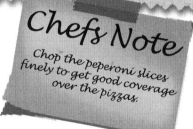

Chefs Note

Chop the peperoni slices finely to get good coverage over the pizzas.

Hawaiian Pizza

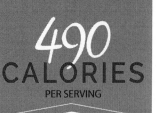

490 CALORIES PER SERVING

Ingredients   Makes 2 Pizzas

2 homemade pizza bases (see page 38 for recipe)

6 tbsp tomato puree/paste

2 garlic cloves, crushed

175g/6oz pineapple chunks

125g/4oz grated low fat mozzarella cheese

100g/3½oz cooked ham, roughly chopped

Salt & pepper to taste

1. Preheat the oven to 220C/450F/Gas Mark 8 and roll out the pizza bases.

2. Mix together the tomato puree & garlic and spread it evenly over the two bases. Add the pineapple, grated cheese and chopped ham.

3. Place in the oven and cook for 8-12 minutes or until golden brown, cooked through and piping hot.

Chefs Note
Pineapple & ham is a takeaway favourite. Add some onions or mushrooms if you like.

Spicy Beef Pizza

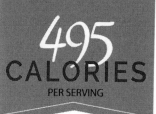

495 CALORIES PER SERVING

Ingredients   Makes 2 Pizzas

2 homemade pizza bases (see page 38 for recipe)
100g/3oz lean minced beef
1 tbsp dried oregano
1 tsp chilli powder
120ml/½ cup beef stock
5 tbsp tomato puree/paste
2 garlic cloves, crushed

1 red chilli, deseeded & finely sliced
1 onion, chopped
50g/2oz grated low fat mozzarella cheese
Low cal cooking oil spray
Salt & pepper to taste

1. Preheat the oven to 220C/450F/Gas Mark 8 and roll out the pizza bases.

2. Quickly brown the beef mince in a frying pan for a few minutes. Add the oregano, chilli powder and beef stock and cook on a high heat for a minute or two until the stock reduces.

3. Place in a food processor and pulse for a few seconds to separate the beef and make it easier to 'crumble' over the pizza.

4. Mix together the tomato puree & garlic and spread it evenly over the two bases. Add the beef, sliced chilli & onion to the pizzas. Lastly sprinkle over the grated cheese.

5. Place in the oven and cook for 8-12 minutes or until golden brown, cooked through and piping hot.

Chefs Note
You could try using turkey mince for this recipe as an even leaner alternative.

Margherita Pizza

Ingredients   Makes 2 Pizzas

2 homemade pizza bases (see page 38 for recipe)
300g/1oz ripe plum tomatoes, chopped
1 tbsp dried basil
2 garlic cloves, crushed

6 tbsp tomato puree/paste
125g/4oz grated low fat mozzarella cheese
Salt & pepper to taste

Chefs Note
This classic pizza is great served with a rocket leaf salad.

1. Preheat the oven to 220C/450F/Gas Mark 8 and roll out the pizza bases.

2. Mix together the chopped tomatoes, basil & garlic. Spread the tomato puree evenly over the two bases. Add the chopped tomatoes mix along with the grated mozzarella.

3. Place in the oven and cook for 8-12 minutes or until golden brown, cooked through and piping hot.

Florentine Pizza

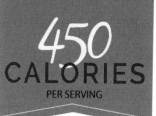

450 CALORIES PER SERVING

Ingredients   Makes 2 Pizzas

2 homemade pizza bases (see page 38 for recipe)
200g/7oz ripe plum tomatoes, chopped
1 tbsp dried basil
2 garlic cloves, crushed
6 tbsp tomato puree/paste
150g/5oz spinach leaves

150g/5oz mushrooms, sliced
2 tbsp grated Parmesan cheese
2 free-range eggs, whites only
Salt & pepper to taste

1. Preheat the oven to 220C/450F/Gas Mark 8 and roll out the pizza bases.

2. Mix together the chopped tomatoes, basil & garlic. Spread the tomato puree evenly over the two bases.

3. Add the spinach and mushrooms to a pan with a splash of boiling water and cook for 2 minutes or until the spinach wilts.

4. Spread the wilted spinach, mushrooms & grated Parmesan over the two bases. Make a well in the centre of each pizza and break in the egg whites.

5. Place in the oven and cook for 8-12 minutes or until golden brown, cooked through and piping hot.

Chefs Note
A little rocket makes a good garnish for this pizza.

Mushroom & Green Pepper Pizza

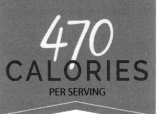

470 CALORIES PER SERVING

Ingredients   Makes 2 Pizzas

2 homemade pizza bases (see page 38 for recipe)
200g/7oz ripe plum tomatoes, chopped
1 tbsp dried basil
2 garlic cloves, crushed
6 tbsp tomato puree/paste
2 green peppers, deseeded & diced

200g/7oz mushrooms, sliced
50g/2oz grated low fat grated cheddar cheese
Salt & pepper to taste

1. Preheat the oven to 220C/450F/Gas Mark 8 and roll out the pizza bases.

2. Mix together the chopped tomatoes, basil & garlic. Spread the tomato puree evenly over the two bases.

3. Spread the wilted peppers, mushrooms & grated cheese over the two bases.

4. Place in the oven and cook for 8-12 minutes or until golden brown, cooked through and piping hot.

Chefs Note

Use vegetarian cheese to make this a veggie treat.

Olive, Caper & Rocket Pizza

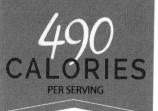
490 CALORIES PER SERVING

Ingredients   Makes 2 Pizzas

2 homemade pizza bases (see page 38 for recipe)

200g/7oz ripe plum tomatoes, chopped

1 tbsp dried basil

2 garlic cloves, crushed

6 tbsp tomato puree/paste

2 tbsp black pitted olives, sliced

1 tbsp capers, rinsed & chopped

125g/4oz grated low fat mozzarella cheese

50g/2oz rocket

Salt & pepper to taste

1. Preheat the oven to 220C/450F/Gas Mark 8 and roll out the pizza bases.

2. Mix together the chopped tomatoes, basil & garlic. Spread the tomato puree evenly over the two bases.

3. Spread the olives, capers & grated cheese over the two bases.

4. Place in the oven and cook for 8-12 minutes or until golden brown, cooked through and piping hot. Sprinkle over the rocket and serve.

Chefs Note

For something different try using sundried tomato puree in place of regular puree.

Dough Balls

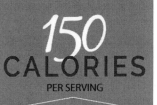
Ingredients   Serves 4

2.5g/¾ tsp dried yeast
165g/5½oz strong white bread flour
Pinch of salt

Pinch of caster sugar
120ml/½ cup warm water

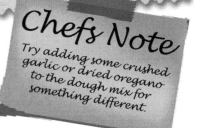

Chefs Note
Try adding some crushed garlic or dried oregano to the dough mix for something different.

1. Combine all the ingredients together by hand or use a mixer. Work the ingredients until the dough comes together to form a ball. Use your hands to knead the dough well on a floured surface for about 8 minutes until it becomes soft and springy. Place the dough in a bowl, cover with cling film and leave to rest at room temperature for 15 minutes. After this time split the dough into approx. 12 small dough balls by rolling in your hands.

2. Brush the dough balls with a little milk or egg white and place on a baking tray in a preheated oven at 200C/400F/Gas Mark 7 for 8-12 minutes or until cooked through and piping hot.

Garlic bread

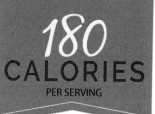
Ingredients   Serves 4

2.5g/¾ tsp dried yeast
165g/5½oz strong white bread flour
Large pinch of salt
Large pinch of caster sugar

120ml/½ cup warm water
1 tsp runny honey
1 tbsp olive oil
4 garlic cloves, crushed

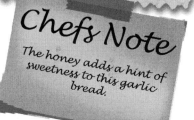

Chefs Note

The honey adds a hint of sweetness to this garlic bread.

1. Combine all the ingredients together by hand or use a mixer. Work the ingredients until the dough comes together to form a ball. Use your hands to knead the dough well on a floured surface for about 8 minutes until it becomes soft and springy. Place the dough in a bowl, cover with cling film and leave to rest at room temperature for 15 minutes. After this time split the dough in half and roll out into two thin bases. The thinner the better.

2. Mix together the honey & olive oil and brush over each base evenly. Cook in a preheated oven at 220C/450F/Gas Mark 8 for 6-9 minutes or until cooked through and piping hot. Brush the crushed garlic over the cooked bases and cook for just a minute or two longer. (You don't want the garlic to brown and crisp up).

Bruschetta

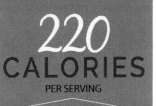

220 CALORIES PER SERVING

Ingredients   Serves 4

2.5g/¾ tsp dried yeast
165g/5½oz strong white bread flour
Large pinch of salt
Large pinch of caster sugar
120ml/½ cup warm water
1 tsp dried oregano or basil
1 tbsp olive oil

200g/7oz ripe plum tomatoes, finely chopped
½ red onion, finely chopped
Salt & pepper to taste

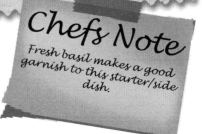

Chefs Note
Fresh basil makes a good garnish to this starter/side dish.

1. Combine the yeast, flour, salt, sugar & water together by hand or use a mixer. Work the ingredients until the dough comes together to form a ball. Use your hands to knead the dough well on a floured surface for about 8 minutes until it becomes soft and springy. Place the dough in a bowl, cover with cling film and leave to rest at room temperature for 15 minutes. After this time split the dough into four and roll out into four even bases. Lightly brush with a little of the olive oil.

2. Cook in a preheated oven at 220C/450F/Gas Mark 8 for 6-9 minutes or until cooked through and piping hot.

3. Mix together the dried herbs, olive oil, tomatoes & red onion and divide across the cooked bases. Season well and serve.

Skinny

SOUTHERN STYLE
& SPICED CHICKEN

'Fried' Chicken On The Bone

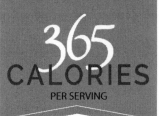

365 CALORIES PER SERVING

Ingredients   Serves 2

4 skinless chicken thighs
250ml/1 cup low fat buttermilk
2 tbsp plain flour
½ tsp each salt, pepper, garlic powder & celery salt
2 tsp paprika
20g/1oz low fat 'butter' spread
200g/7oz mixed salad leaves
200g/7oz plum tomatoes, sliced
1 red onion, sliced
Salt & pepper to taste

1. Preheat the oven to 200c/400f/gas mark 6.

2. Pierce the chicken thighs with a fork a few times and place in a bowl with the buttermilk. Combine really well, cover and leave to marinade for a few hours if possible (don't worry if you don't have time even half an hour is worth it).

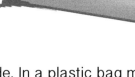

Chefs Note
Baking, rather than deep-frying, is a much healthier alternative.

3. Take the thighs out of the buttermilk and put to one side. In a plastic bag mix together the flour, salt, pepper, garlic powder, celery salt & paprika.

4. Place the thighs in the flour bag and coat thoroughly.

5. Heat the 'butter' spread in a large saucepan and place the chicken in the hot pan. Cook for 1-2 minutes until browned (don't move the chicken around as the coating will fall off). Turn the chicken over and cook for 1-2 minutes longer until browned on both sides.

6. Carefully transfer the chicken to a rack on a baking tray and place in the preheated oven. Put on the top shelf and cook for 20-30 minutes or until the chicken is crispy and cooked through.

7. Serve with the tomatoes & red onion salad.

Hot Wings

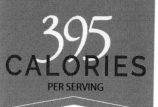
Ingredients Serves 2

12 skinless chicken wings
250ml/1 cup low fat buttermilk
2 tbsp plain flour
1 tsp each ground black pepper,
cayenne pepper & garlic powder
½ tsp salt
20g/1oz low fat 'butter' spread
3 tbsp fat free Greek yoghurt

2 tbsp freshly chopped chives
Salt & pepper to taste

1. Preheat the oven to 200c/400f/gas mark 6.

2. Pierce the chicken wings with a fork a few times and place in a bowl with the buttermilk. Combine really well, cover and leave to marinade for a few hours if possible (don't worry if you don't have time even half an hour is worth it).

Chefs Note

Adjust the cayenne pepper in this recipe to suit your own taste.

3. Take the wings out of the buttermilk and put to one side.

4. In a plastic bag mix together the flour, black pepper, cayenne pepper, garlic powder & salt. Place the wings in the flour bag and coat thoroughly.

5. Heat the 'butter' spread in a large saucepan and place the chicken in the hot pan. Cook for 1-2 minutes until browned (don't move the chicken around as the coating will fall off). Turn the wings over and cook for 1-2 minutes longer until browned on both sides. Carefully transfer the chicken to a rack on a baking tray and place in the preheated oven. Put on the top shelf and cook for 15-25 minutes or until the wings are crispy and cooked through.

6. Mix the Greek yoghurt and chives together to make a cooling dip and serve on the side with the chicken wings.

Boneless 'Fried' Chicken Strips

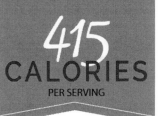
Ingredients   Serves 2

400g/14oz skinless chicken breasts
250ml/1 cup low fat buttermilk
2 tbsp plain flour
½ tsp each salt, pepper, garlic powder &
celery salt

2 tsp paprika
20g/1oz low fat 'butter' spread
Salt & pepper to taste

1. Preheat the oven to 200c/400f/gas mark 6.

2. Cut the chicken breast into thick strips about 2-3cm wide and place in a bowl with the buttermilk. Combine really well, cover and leave to marinade for a few hours if possible (don't worry if you don't have time even half an hour is worth it).

3. Take the strips out of the buttermilk and put to one side. In a plastic bag mix together the flour, salt, pepper, garlic powder, celery salt & paprika.

4. Place the strips in the flour bag and coat thoroughly.

5. Heat the 'butter' spread in a large saucepan and place the chicken strips in the hot pan. Cook for 1-2 minutes until browned (don't move the chicken around as the coating will fall off). Turn the chicken over and cook for 1-2 minutes longer until browned on both sides.

6. Carefully transfer the chicken strips to a rack on a baking tray and place in the preheated oven. Put on the top shelf and cook for 10-20 minutes or until the chicken is crispy and cooked through.

Chefs Note
This is lovely served with homemade low fat coleslaw.

Popcorn Chicken With BBQ Sauce

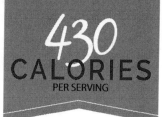

430 CALORIES PER SERVING

Ingredients   Serves 2

400g/14oz free-range skinless chicken breasts
250ml/1 cup low fat buttermilk
2 tbsp plain flour
½ tsp each salt, pepper, garlic powder & celery salt
2 tsp paprika
20g/1oz low fat 'butter' spread

3 tbsp ketchup
1 tbsp Worcestershire sauce
1 tbsp cider vinegar
1 tsp caster sugar
Salt & pepper to taste

1. Preheat the oven to 200c/400f/gas mark 6.

2. Cube the chicken breast into equal sized pieces and place in a bowl with the buttermilk. Combine really well, cover and leave to marinade for a few hours if possible (don't worry if you don't have time even half an hour is worth it).

3. Take the chicken out of the buttermilk and put to one side.

4. In a plastic bag mix together the flour, salt, pepper, garlic powder, celery salt & paprika. Place the chicken in the flour bag and coat thoroughly.

5. Heat the 'butter' spread in a large saucepan and place the chicken in the hot pan. Cook for 1-2 minutes on each side on a high heat (don't move the chicken around as the coating will fall off). Carefully transfer the chicken to a rack on a baking tray and place in the preheated oven. Put on the top shelf and cook for 8-15 minutes or until the chicken is crispy and cooked through.

6. Meanwhile mix together the ketchup, Worcestershire sauce, vinegar and sugar to make a simple BBQ sauce. Serve on the side with the cooked popcorn chicken.

Chefs Note
Adjust the cooking time depending on how big you cube your chicken.

Homemade Coleslaw

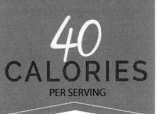

40 CALORIES
PER SERVING

Ingredients   Serves 4

2 carrots
½ white cabbage
1 bunch spring onions
1 tbsp low fat mayonnaise

4 tbsp fat free Greek yoghurt
1 tsp Dijon mustard
Salt & pepper to taste

1. Use a vegetable peeler to slice the carrots into julienne ribbons.

2. Finely shred the cabbage and thinly slice the spring onions.

3. Mix together the mayonnaise, yoghurt & mustard and combine with the chopped vegetables. Season and serve.

Chefs Note

You could also add a little lemon juice to this fresh crunchy coleslaw if you like.

Breaded Chicken Burger

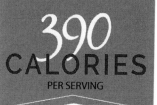

Ingredients   Serves 4

4 free-range skinless chicken breasts each weighing 125g/4oz
2 slices bread
1 tsp garlic powder
½ tsp salt
1 free-range egg
1 baby gem lettuce shredded
1 tbsp low fat mayonnaise

4 regular brown burger rolls
Salt & pepper to taste

Chefs Note

Toasted breadcrumbs makes a crispier coating but you can use untoasted too.

1. Preheat the oven grill.

2. Bash the chicken breasts with a meat hammer for a few seconds until their thickness is reduced by about half.

3. Toast the bread and place in a food processor with the garlic powder and salt to make crunchy breadcrumbs. Spread the breadcrumbs out evenly on a plate.

4. Lightly beat the egg in a bowl and dip the flattened chicken breasts in turn into the egg. Press the egg-covered Chicken breasts hard onto the breadcrumbs until completely coated in breadcrumbs.

5. Place the breaded chicken breasts on a rack under the grill and cook for 4-5 minutes each side or until the chicken is cooked through.

6. Spread the rolls with the mayonnaise and serve the cooked chicken and shredded lettuce inside.

Grilled BBQ Chicken Burger

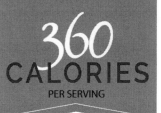
360 CALORIES PER SERVING

Ingredients   Serves 4

4 free-range skinless chicken breasts each weighing 125g/4oz

1 tbsp runny honey

3 tbsp ketchup

1 tbsp Worcestershire sauce

1 tbsp cider vinegar

1 tsp caster sugar

2 large beef tomatoes, sliced

1 baby gem lettuce shredded

4 regular brown burger rolls

Salt & pepper to taste

Chefs Note

Brushing the chicken breasts with honey gives the burger a lovely sweetness.

1. Preheat the oven grill.

2. Bash the chicken breasts with a meat hammer for a few seconds so that the breasts are the same thickness throughout.

3. Lightly brush each side of the chicken breast with honey and place on a rack under the grill. Cook for 5-8 minutes each side or until the chicken is cooked through.

4. Mix together the ketchup, Worcestershire sauce, vinegar and sugar to make the BBQ sauce.

5. Spread the rolls with the BBQ sauce and serve the cooked chicken, shredded lettuce & sliced tomatoes inside.

Chicken Tikka Wrap

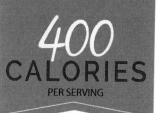

400 CALORIES PER SERVING

Ingredients   Serves 4

500g/1lb 2oz free-range skinless chicken breasts, cubed
3 tbsp fat free Greek yoghurt
1 tbsp curry powder
2 garlic cloves, crushed
2 large beef tomatoes, chopped
1 baby gem lettuce shredded
4 low fat tortilla wraps

Low cal cooking oil spray
Salt & pepper to taste

1. Season the chicken and pierce with a fork so that the chicken can 'take on' the marinade.

2. Mix together the yoghurt, curry powder and garlic and add the cubed chicken to a large bowl. Combine well, cover and leave to marinade for a few hours (if you have time).

3. Preheat the oven grill.

4. Spray with a little low cal oil and place the marinated chicken on a rack under the grill. Cook for 3-6 minutes each side or until the chicken is cooked through.

5. Serve the cooked chicken along with the chopped tomatoes & lettuce rolled up in the wraps. Cut in half and serve.

Chefs Note

Serving with lemon wedges gives a welcome citrus twist to this recipe.

Cajun Corn

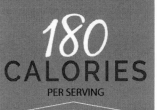

Ingredients   Serves 4

2 tbsp olive oil

1 tsp each paprika & garlic powder

½ tsp salt

2 tsp Tabasco sauce (or to taste)

4 large sweetcorn cobs, husks removed

Salt & pepper to taste

1. Preheat the grill.

2. Mix together the oil, paprika, powder, salt & Tabasco sauce.

3. Brush the corn with the spiced oil and place under the grill. Place under a medium heat and, turning occasionally, cook for 10-14 minutes or until tender and cooked through.

Chefs Note

Corn on the cob is traditionally dripping with butter. This lower fat Cajun version is a crunchy healthier alterative.

Piri Piri Chicken On The Bone

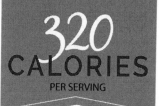

320 CALORIES PER SERVING

Ingredients   Serves 2

2 garlic cloves
2 birds eye chillies, deseeded
1 tbsp each paprika & Worcestershire sauce
1 tsp each salt & dried oregano
1 tbsp olive oil

4 skinless chicken thighs
4 tbsp fat free Greek yoghurt
Salt & pepper to taste

1. Preheat the grill.

2. Place the chillies, paprika, Worcestershire sauce, salt, oregano & oil in a blender and whizz to a smooth consistency to make a sauce (add a little water if the sauce needs loosening up).

Chefs Note

This chicken is HOT! For extra spice don't deseed the chillies.

3. Brush chicken thighs with the hot sauce. Place on a rack on under the grill and cook for 20-25 minutes or until the chicken is cooked through.

4. Serve with a spoonful of cool yoghurt for dipping.

Piri Piri Butterfly Burger

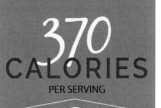

370 CALORIES PER SERVING

Ingredients   Serves 4

4 free-range skinless chicken breasts each weighing 125g/4oz
2 garlic cloves
2 birds eye chillies, deseeded
1 tbsp each paprika & Worcestershire sauce
1 tsp each salt & dried oregano
1 tbsp olive oil
2 large beef tomatoes, sliced

1 baby gem lettuce shredded
4 regular brown burger rolls
Salt & pepper to taste

Chefs Note
The butterflied breast chicken should cook quickly so make sure you don't overcook.

1. Preheat the grill.

2. Butterfly the chicken by laying the breast on a flat surface. Use a sharp knife to cut along the long side of the breast. Slice through until you have almost cut the breast right through. Open up the butterfly by folding out the breast into two joined halves.

3. Place the chillies, paprika, Worcestershire sauce, salt, oregano & oil in a blender and whizz to a smooth consistency to make a sauce (add a little water if the sauce needs loosening up).

4. Brush butterflied breasts on both sides with the hot sauce. Place on a rack on under the grill and cook for 8-12 minutes or until the chicken is cooked through.

5. Lightly toast the burger rolls and serve with the chicken, shredded lettuce & sliced tomatoes inside.

Piri Piri Pitta

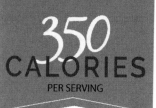

350 CALORIES PER SERVING

Ingredients
Serves 4

500g/1lb 2oz free-range skinless chicken breasts
2 garlic cloves
2 birds eye chillies, deseeded
1 tbsp each paprika & Worcestershire sauce
1 tsp each salt & dried oregano
1 tbsp olive oil

2 large beef tomatoes, chopped
1 red onion, sliced
2 tbsp fat free Greek yogurt
4 regular pitta breads
Salt & pepper to taste

1. Preheat the grill.

2. Slice the chicken into thick strips.

3. Place the chillies, paprika, Worcestershire sauce, salt, oregano & oil in a blender and whizz to a smooth consistency to make a sauce (add a little water if the sauce needs loosening up).

4. Combine the sauce and chicken strips together. Lay out on a rack under the grill and cook for 4-6 minutes or until the chicken is cooked through.

5. Lightly warm the pitta bread and open into pockets.

6. Load the pitta pockets with the cooked chicken, chopped tomatoes and sliced onion with a dollop of yoghurt on top.

Chefs Note
Fresh red onion gives this dish a lovely crunch. Add a dash of lemon juice if you like.

Piri Piri Veggie Burger

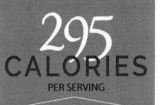
Ingredients   Serves 4

400g/14oz tinned chickpeas, drained
1 free-range egg
2 garlic cloves
2 birds eye chillies, deseeded & finely chopped
1 tbsp each paprika & Worcestershire sauce
1 tsp each salt & dried oregano
1 tbsp olive oil

1 tbsp lemon juice
2 large beef tomatoes, sliced
1 baby gem lettuce shredded
4 regular white burger rolls
Salt & pepper to taste

Chefs Note
Use a plastic burger mould if you can. They are very cheap and really improve the texture of the burger.

1. Preheat the grill.

2. Place the chickpeas, egg, garlic, chillies, paprika, Worcestershire sauce, salt, oregano, oil and lemon juice in a food processor and whizz to a chunky consistency.

3. Form the mixture into four burger patties. Place on a rack under the grill and cook for 8-12 minutes or until cooked through and piping hot.

4. Lightly toast the burger rolls and serve with the chickpea burgers, shredded lettuce & sliced tomatoes inside.

Skinny
BURGERS

Classic Cheese Burger With Fresh Relish

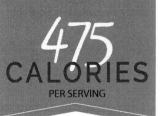

475 CALORIES PER SERVING

Ingredients
Serves 4

500g/1lb 2oz lean mince beef
2 tsp Worcestershire sauce
½ onion, finely chopped
3 garlic cloves, crushed
½ tsp salt
1 whole serving of fresh burger relish (see page 68 for recipe)
1 large beef tomatoes, sliced

1 baby gem lettuce shredded
4 slices low fat cheddar cheese
4 regular brown burger rolls
Low cal cooking oil spray
Salt & pepper to taste

1. Preheat the grill.

2. Place the beef, Worcestershire sauce, onion, garlic & salt in a food processor and pulse a few times to combine well.

3. Form the mixture into four burger patties. Spray with a little low cal oil. Place on a rack under the grill and cook for 8-12 minutes or until cooked through and piping hot.

4. Lightly toast the burger rolls and spread with the burger relish. Serve with the burgers, shredded lettuce & sliced tomatoes inside.

Chefs Note
Sometimes only a burger will hit the spot! Use a plastic burger mould to get the best texture.

Hot Jerk Burger With Grilled Pineapple

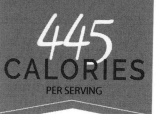

445 CALORIES PER SERVING

Ingredients   Serves 4

500g/1lb 2oz lean mince beef
½ onion, finely chopped
1 garlic clove, crushed
½ tsp each salt, cinnamon, allspice & nutmeg
1 tsp each ground coriander, ginger & chilli powder
4 tinned pineapple rings, drained
1 baby gem lettuce shredded
4 regular white burger rolls
Lime wedges to serve
Low cal cooking oil spray
Salt & pepper to taste

1. Preheat the grill.

2. Place the beef, onion, garlic, and dried spices in a food processor and pulse a few times to combine well.

Chefs Note
It's fine to use a shop bought jerk seasoning if that's what's you have you hand.

3. If you have one, use a plastic burger mould to form the mixture into four burger patties and spray with a little low cal oil.

4. Place the burgers and the pineapple rings on a rack under the grill and cook for 8-12 minutes or until everything is cooked through and piping hot.

5. Lightly toast the burger rolls and serve with the burgers, shredded lettuce & pineapple slice inside and the lime wedges on the side.

Kofta Burger

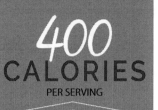

400 CALORIES
PER SERVING

Ingredients   Serves 4

500g/1lb 2oz extra lean minced lamb
½ onion, finely chopped
3 garlic cloves, crushed
1 tbsp medium or hot curry powder
½ tsp salt
1 baby gem lettuce shredded
4 regular pitta bread

2 tbsp fat free Greek yoghurt
Low cal cooking oil spray
Salt & pepper to taste

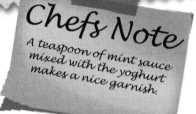

Chefs Note
A teaspoon of mint sauce mixed with the yoghurt makes a nice garnish.

1. Preheat the grill.

2. Place the lamb, onion, garlic, curry powder & salt in a food processor and pulse a few times to combine well.

3. If you have a plastic burger mould use it to form the mixture into four burger patties (or use your hands) and spray with a little low cal oil.

4. Place the burgers on a rack under the grill and cook for 8-12 minutes or until everything is cooked through and piping hot.

5. Lightly warm the pitta bread and open them up into pockets. Serve with the burgers, and shredded lettuce inside with a dollop of yoghurt on top.

Spicy Bean Burger With Tabasco Mayonnaise

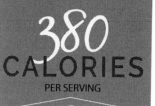

380 CALORIES PER SERVING

Ingredients   Serves 4

500g/1lb 2oz tinned mixed beans, drained & rinsed
3 garlic cloves, crushed
1 tsp cayenne pepper
½ tsp each salt & ground coriander
1 tbsp lime juice
1 free-range egg
2 tbsp low fat mayonnaise

Large dash Tabasco sauce
2 large beef tomatoes, sliced
1 red onion, sliced
1 baby gem lettuce shredded
4 regular white burger rolls
Low cal cooking oil spray
Salt & pepper to taste

Chefs Note

Use dried beans if you like, provided they are soaked overnight.

1. Preheat the grill.

2. Place the beans, garlic, cayenne pepper, salt, coriander, lime juice & egg in a food processor and pulse a few times to combine well and break down the beans a little.

3. If you have a plastic burger mould form the mixture into four burger patties (or use your hands) and spray with a little low cal oil.

4. Place the burgers on a rack under the grill and cook for 8-12 minutes or until cooked through and piping hot.

5. Mix together the Tabasco sauce and mayonnaise. Lightly toast the rolls and serve with the burgers, sliced tomatoes, red onion & shredded lettuce inside along with the Tabasco mayonnaise on top.

Fresh Burger Relish

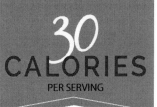

30 CALORIES PER SERVING

Ingredients Serves 4

400g/14oz ripe plum tomatoes
1 tbsp tomato puree
1 tsp each paprika, salt & brown sugar

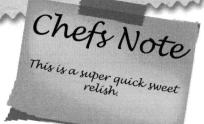

Chefs Note

This is a super quick sweet relish.

1. Place all the ingredients in a food processor and pulse until the tomatoes are finely chopped and everything has combined to form a fresh relish.

2. Check the balance of spice, salt & sugar and adjust if needed. Serve loaded on top of your favourite burger.

Spicy Plum Tomato Relish

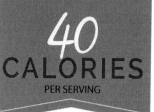

Ingredients   Serves 4

400g/14oz ripe plum tomatoes
1 tsp cumin
2 garlic cloves
1 stick celery
1 tbsp tomato puree

1 red chilli, deseeded & chopped
1 tsp each paprika, salt & brown sugar
Low cal cooking oil spray

1. Place all the ingredients in a food processor and pulse until the tomatoes are finely chopped and everything has combined.

2. Heat a little low cal oil in a frying pan and gently cook for 15-25 minutes or until the relish is cooked and combined. Allow to cool, refrigerate and serve with burgers.

Chefs Note

Use crushed chilli flakes if you don't have fresh chillies to hand.

Sweet-Sweetcorn Relish

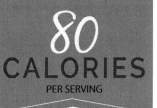

80 CALORIES
PER SERVING

Ingredients   Serves 4

1 onion, sliced
300g/11oz tinned sweetcorn, drained
1 tsp ground coriander
1 red pepper, deseeded & diced
2 garlic cloves
2 tsp brown sugar

1 tbsp cider vinegar
½ tsp salt
Low cal cooking oil spray

1. Heat a little low cal oil in a frying pan and gently cook all the ingredients for 25-30 minutes or until the sweetcorn is cooked and syrupy.

2. Allow to cool, refrigerate and serve with burgers.

Chefs Note
Add a little more sugar if you feel the relish needs it.

Sweet Potato Fries

Ingredients   Serves 4

600g/1lb 5oz sweet potatoes
1 tbsp olive oil
½ tsp salt flakes

1. Preheat the oven to 180c/350f/gas mark 4.

2. Peel the sweet potatoes and cut into thin fries. Square of the ends to prevent burning while cooking.

3. Combine well in a bowl with the olive oil and salt, making sure every chip is coated with oil.

4. Place the fries on a baking tray in the preheated oven and cook for 20-30 minutes or until the fries are crispy and golden.

5. Season and serve.

Chefs Note
Sweet potatoes are tasty alternative to regular potatoes.

Lighter Potato Salad

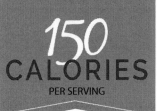

Ingredients   Serves 4

500g/1lb 2oz salad potatoes
2 tbsp low fat crème fraiche
2 tsp Dijon mustard

Bunch fresh chives, shopped
Salt & pepper to taste
1 tbsp olive oil

1. Cut the salad potatoes in half and cook for 8-10 minutes in salted boiling water or until tender.

2. Drain and allow to cool for a few minutes.

3. Mix together the creme fraiche, mustard & chives and combine with the warm potatoes.

4. Season with lots of black pepper, chill & serve.

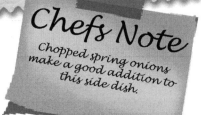

Chefs Note

Chopped spring onions make a good addition to this side dish.

Chunky Chips

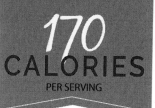

170 CALORIES PER SERVING

Ingredients Serves 4

600g/1lb 5oz potatoes
1 tbsp olive oil
Salt & pepper to taste

1. Preheat the oven to 220c/450f/gas mark 8.

2. Peel the potatoes and cut into thick chips about 1cm square.

3. Plunge into a pan of boiling unsalted water and cook for 3 minutes. Drain and quickly dry off with kitchen towel.

4. Place the blanched chips in a bowl with the olive oil & seasoning. Combine really well making sure every chip is coated with oil.

5. Place the chips on a baking tray in the preheated oven and cook for approx. 15 minutes or until the fries are crispy and golden on the outside and tender on the inside.

6. Season and serve.

Chefs Note

Oven baked chunky chips are a far heather alternative to deep-fried fries.

Skinny
MEXICAN

Beef Burrito

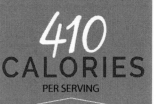

410 CALORIES PER SERVING

Ingredients   Serves 4

500g/1lb 2oz lean beef mince

2 garlic cloves, crushed

1 onion, sliced

1 red chilli, deseeded & finely chopped

1 tsp each ground coriander, cumin & paprika

200g/7oz ripe plum tomatoes, finely chopped

1 romaine lettuce shredded

2 tbsp fat free Greek yoghurt

4 soft flour low fat tortillas

Salt & pepper to taste

Chefs Note

Regular burritos usual contain heavy grated cheese and rice.

1. Quickly brown the mince for a minute or two along with the garlic cloves, onion & chillies. Add the coriander, cumin & paprika and cook for 4-6 minutes until the beef is cooked through.

2. Remove from the heat, stir through the chopped tomatoes and pile into the flour tortillas. Add lettuce and yoghurt, roll and serve.

Turkey Tacos

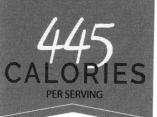

445 CALORIES PER SERVING

Ingredients
Serves 4

500g/1lb 2oz lean turkey mince

200g/7oz ripe plum tomatoes, finely chopped

2 garlic cloves, crushed

1 onion, sliced

2 tsp each cumin & paprika

100g/3½oz low gat grated cheddar cheese

1 romaine lettuce shredded

4 taco shells

Salt & pepper to taste

1. Quickly brown the turkey mince for a minute or two. Add the plum tomatoes, garlic, onions, cumin & paprika and cook for a few minutes until the turkey is cooked through and the onions are tender.

2. Remove from the heat and pile into the taco shells with the lettuce underneath and the grated cheese on top.

3. Serve immediately.

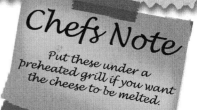

Chefs Note

Put these under a preheated grill if you want the cheese to be melted.

Chicken Fajitas

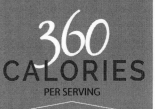

360 CALORIES PER SERVING

Ingredients   Serves 4

500g/1lb 2oz skinless free-range chicken breasts

2 garlic cloves, crushed

1 tsp each cumin, coriander & paprika

2 red peppers, deseeded & sliced

1 red chilli, deseeded & finely chopped

1 onion, sliced

1 tbsp lime juice

2 baby gem lettuces, shredded

4 soft flour low fat tortillas

200g/7oz ripe plum tomatoes, chopped

1 tbsp olive oil

Salt & pepper to taste

Chefs Note
Sliced steak also works really well in these fajitas.

1. Slice the chicken breasts into strips and combine well with the garlic, cumin, coriander & paprika.

2. Heat the olive oil in a frying pan and gently saute the peppers, chilli and onions for a few minutes until softened. Add the chicken and cook for 5-7 minutes or until the chicken strips are cooked through. Stir through the lime, remove from the heat and pile into the flour tortillas with the shredded lettuce and chopped tomatoes.

Chunky Fresh Guacamole

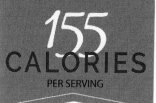

Ingredients   Serves 4

2 ripe avocados
1 ripe plum tomato
½ red onion
½ tsp chilli powder (or more to taste)

2 tbsp lime juice
3 tbsp freshly chopped coriander
Salt & pepper to taste

1. De-stone and peel the avocados. Dice into small cubes and put in a bowl.

2. Finely chop the tomato and onions. Add to the bowl along with the chilli powder, lime, chopped coriander and plenty of salt & pepper.

3. Combine well, using the back of a fork now and again to crush some of the avocado. This will give the guacamole a chunky feel but will bring the sauce together a little.

Chefs Note
You can blend this to a smooth consistency in the food processor if you prefer.

Simple Salsa

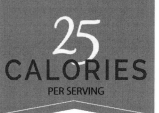

25
CALORIES
PER SERVING

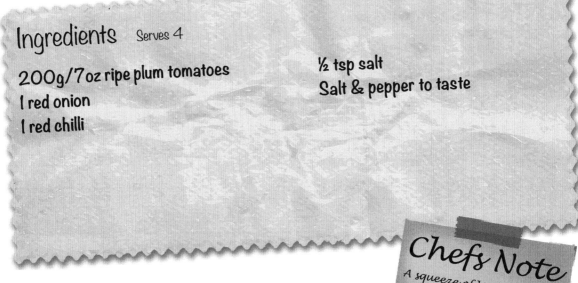

Ingredients   Serves 4

200g/7oz ripe plum tomatoes
1 red onion
1 red chilli

½ tsp salt
Salt & pepper to taste

1. Dice the plum tomatoes and red onion. Deseed the chilli and chop finely. Combine everything together in a bowl with the salt.

2. Check the seasoning and serve.

Chefs Note

A squeeze of lime juice and some chopped coriander make good additions to this simple salsa.

Lighter Nachos

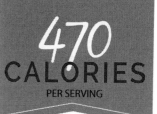

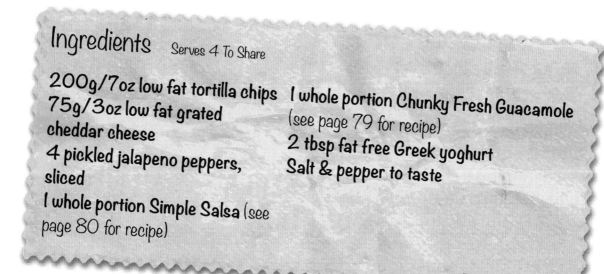

Ingredients   Serves 4 To Share

200g/7oz low fat tortilla chips
75g/3oz low fat grated cheddar cheese
4 pickled jalapeno peppers, sliced
1 whole portion Simple Salsa (see page 80 for recipe)

1 whole portion Chunky Fresh Guacamole (see page 79 for recipe)
2 tbsp fat free Greek yoghurt
Salt & pepper to taste

1. Preheat the grill.

2. Place the tortilla chips on a large ovenproof plate. Arrange the grated cheese and sliced jalapeno peppers on top and cook under the grill for a few minutes until the cheese melts.

3. Load the salsa, guacamole & yoghurt into three mounds evenly spaced around the plate of tortilla chips. Season and serve.

Chefs Note

Nachos are notoriously calorific. This skinny version helps keep the calories down.

Mexican Ceviche

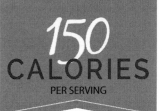

150 CALORIES PER SERVING

Ingredients   Serves 4

500g/1lb 2oz skinless, boneless white fish fillet

120ml/ ½ cup fresh lime juice

1 large bunch spring onions, finely chopped

1 green chilli, deseeded & finely chopped

½ tsp cayenne pepper

1 large beef tomato, finely diced

½ tsp brown sugar

4 tbsp freshly chopped coriander

Salt & pepper to taste

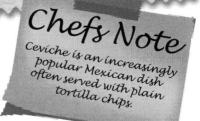

Chefs Note

Ceviche is an increasingly popular Mexican dish often served with plain tortilla chips.

1. Slice the fish into thin strips. In a bowl combine the fish strips, lime juice & spring onions.

2. Cover and leave to chill for 2 hours. After this time drain the juice from the fish and onions and combine with the rest of the ingredients.

3. Check the seasoning and serve.

Mexican Rice

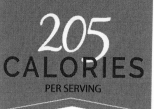

205
CALORIES
PER SERVING

Ingredients   Serves 4

200g/7oz rice
1 chicken stock cube
1 whole portion Simple Salsa (see page 80 for recipe)
Salt & pepper to taste

1. Cook the rice in a pan of boiling salted water with the stock cube crumbled in.

2. When the rice is tender drain and add to a bowl. Stir through the fresh salsa, season and serve immediately.

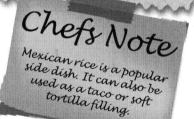

Chefs Note

Mexican rice is a popular side dish. It can also be used as a taco or soft tortilla filling.

Buffalo Wings

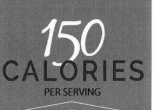

Ingredients   Serves 4

4 garlic cloves, crushed

1 tbsp each Worcestershire sauce & runny honey

1 tsp each paprika, ground black pepper & cayenne pepper

½ tsp salt

12 free-range skinless chicken wings

Salt & pepper to taste

Chefs Note
This delicious spiced side dish can be served hot or cold.

1. Mix together all the ingredients, except the chicken wings, to make a marinade.

2. Pierce the chicken wings with a fork a few times and place in the marinade bowl. Combine really well, cover and leave for a few hours if possible (don't worry if you don't have time even half an hour is worth it).

3. Preheat the oven to 180c/350f/gas mark 6.

4. Transfer the chicken to a rack on a baking tray, place in the preheated oven and cook for 20-30 minutes or until the wings are cooked through.

Light Calamares

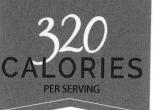

320 CALORIES PER SERVING

Ingredients

Serves 4

3 tbsp plain flour
1 tsp each salt & black pepper
1 tsp paprika
500g/1lb 2oz prepared fresh squid rings
2 free range eggs
150g/5oz panko breadcrumbs
Low cal cooking oil spray

1. Preheat the oven to 200c/400f/gas mark 7.

2. Mix together the flour, salt, pepper & paprika in a large bowl.

Chefs Note
Panko breadcrumbs are readily available in most supermarkets.

3. Make sure the squid is free of excess liquid and combine with the flour mixture in a bowl until well coated.

4. Separate the egg yolks and discard. Lightly beat the egg whites and dip the rings into the beaten whites before rolling in the breadcrumbs.

5. Transfer crumb covered squid rings to a rack on a baking tray and spray with a little low cal oil. Place in the preheated oven and cook for 10-15 minutes or until the squid rings are crispy and golden.

Skinny
KEBABS

'Doner' Kebab

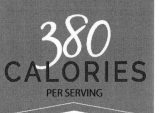

380 CALORIES PER SERVING

Ingredients Serves 2

250g/9oz skinless, chicken breast
250ml/1 cup chicken stock
2 regular pitta bread
2 tbsp fat free Greek yoghurt
1 tsp mint sauce
1 Romaine lettuce, shredded
1 large beef tomatoes, finely sliced

½ red onion sliced
1 tbsp Tabasco sauce
Salt & pepper to taste

Chefs Note
Using chicken in this 'doner' kebab makes for a lower fat alternative to lamb.

1. Place the breasts edge up and slice as thinly as possible through the width of the breast. Season and place in a saucepan with the hot chicken stock. Bring to the boil, reduce the heat and simmer for 4-5 minutes or until the chicken is cooked through.

2. Whilst the chicken is cooking warm the pitta bread under a grill. Combine the yoghurt and mint sauce to make mint yoghurt.

3. Drain the chicken, pat dry of excess stock and load the soft, cooked chicken slices into the pitta bread along with the shredded lettuce, sliced tomatoes, red onions, Tabasco sauce and minted Greek yoghurt.

Veggie Hummus Kebab

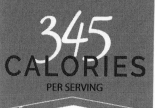

345 CALORIES PER SERVING

Ingredients   Serves 2

200g/7oz tinned chickpeas, drained
½ garlic clove
1 tsp tahini paste
1 tbsp lemon juice
1 tbsp olive oil
½ tsp salt
2 regular pitta bread
2 tbsp fat free Greek yoghurt

1 tsp mint sauce
2 jalapeno peppers, sliced
1 Romaine lettuce, shredded
1 large beef tomatoes, finely sliced
½ red onion sliced
1 tbsp Tabasco sauce
½ cucumber, slice into batons
Salt & pepper to taste

1. Place the chickpeas, garlic, tahini paste, lemon juice, olive oil & salt in a food processor and whizz until smooth.

2. Warm the pitta bread under a grill and combine the yoghurt and mint sauce to make mint yoghurt.

3. Spoon the hummus into the pitta bread along with the jalapeno peppers, shredded lettuce, sliced tomatoes, onions, Tabasco sauce, cucumber and minted Greek yoghurt.

Chefs Note

Balance the lemon juice, garlic and salt to get the hummus just right.

Falafels

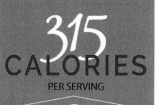

315 CALORIES PER SERVING

Ingredients   Serves 2

200g/7oz tinned chickpeas, drained
½ tsp each ground cumin & coriander
1 free range egg
1 garlic clove, crushed
½ tsp salt
2 regular pitta bread
2 jalapeno peppers, sliced
1 Romaine lettuce, shredded

1 large beef tomatoes, finely sliced
½ red onion sliced
1 tbsp Tabasco sauce
½ cucumber, slice into batons
Low cal cooking oil spray
Salt & pepper to taste

Chefs Note
You could add a little chilli powder to the falafel mixture if you wish.

1. Place the chickpeas, cumin, coriander, egg, garlic & salt in a food processor and pulse to combine.

2. Scoop out the mixture and use your hands to form into small falafel balls.

3. Heat a little low cal cooking oil spray in a frying pan and gently cook the falafels for 6-12 minutes or until cooked through. Meanwhile warm the pitta bread under a grill

4. Place the falafels into the pitta bread along with the jalapeno peppers, shredded lettuce, sliced tomatoes, onions, Tabasco sauce & cucumber.

Lamb Kofta

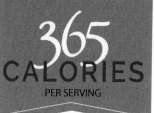

Ingredients   Serves 2

200g/7oz lean lamb mince
½ tsp each ground cumin & coriander
1 garlic clove, crushed
½ tsp salt
2 regular pitta bread
1 baby gem lettuce, shredded
2 tbsp fat free Greek yoghurt

1 tsp mint sauce
4 kebab skewers
Low cal cooking oil spray
Salt & pepper to taste

1. Preheat the grill.

2. Place the lamb mince, cumin, coriander, garlic & salt in a food processor and pulse to combine. Scoop out the mixture and use your hands to form into 4 balls.

3. Roll the balls into oval shapes and thread lengthways onto 4 skewers. Spray with a little low cal oil, place under a preheated medium grill and cook for 5-10 minutes or until cooked through.

4. Mix the yoghurt and mint sauce together.

5. Warm the pitta bread under the grill, take the koftas off the skewers and place in the pittas along with the shredded lettuce & mint yoghurt.

Chefs Note

Try using chicken mince as a leaner alternative if you like.

Chicken Kebab

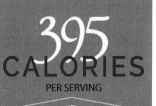

Ingredients   Serves 2

300g/11oz skinless, chicken breast, cubed
½ tsp each ground cumin, coriander, chilli powder & paprika
1 red pepper deseeded & cut into chunks
2 regular pitta bread
1 baby gem lettuce, shredded
2 tbsp fat free Greek yoghurt
1 tsp mint sauce

4 kebab skewers
Low cal cooking oil spray
Salt & pepper to taste

Chefs Note

Add any mix of salad you like to fill out the pittas.

1. Preheat the grill.

2. Season the chicken and combine with the cumin, coriander, chilli powder & paprika.

3. Thread the chicken cubes and red peppers pieces in turn onto the skewers. Spray with a little low cal oil, place under a preheated medium grill and cook for 5-10 minutes or until the chicken is cooked through.

4. Mix the yoghurt and mint sauce together.

5. Warm the pitta bread under the grill. Take the chicken & peppers off the skewers and place in the pittas along with the shredded lettuce & mint yoghurt.

King Prawn Kebab

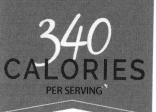

340 CALORIES PER SERVING

Ingredients   Serves 2

300g/11oz raw shelled king prawns
2 garlic cloves, crushed
1 tsp freshly grated ginger
½ tsp coriander & chilli powder
1 red onion, cut into chunks
2 regular pitta bread
1 baby gem lettuce, shredded

2 tbsp fat free Greek yoghurt
1 tsp mint sauce
4 kebab skewers
Lemon wedges to serve
Low cal cooking oil spray
Salt & pepper to taste

1. Preheat the grill.

2. Season the prawns and combine with the garlic, ginger, coriander & chilli powder.

3. Thread the prawns and red onion pieces in turn onto the skewers. Spray with a little low cal oil, place under a preheated medium grill and cook for 4-6 minutes or until the prawns are cooked through.

4. Mix the yoghurt and mint sauce together.

5. Warm the pitta bread under the grill, take the prawns & onions off the skewers and place in the pittas along with the shredded lettuce & mint yoghurt.

6. Serve with lemon wedges.

Chefs Note
If you prefer your red onion softer, cook for a little longer.

Halloumi Pittas

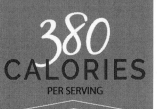

Ingredients   Serves 2

2 regular pitta breads
200g/7oz low fat halloumi cheese, finely sliced
1 red chilli, deseeded & finely chopped

1 baby gem lettuce, shredded
Low cal cooking oil spray
Salt & pepper to taste

Chefs Note
Halloumi cheese pittas are a popular non-meat alternative.

1. Preheat the grill.

2. Split the pitta bread in half to open up into butterflies.

3. Arrange the thinly sliced halloumi and chopped chilli on top on each pitta and place under a medium preheated grill until the cheese begins to brown.

4. Fold each pitta back together takeaway style, load in the lettuce and serve.

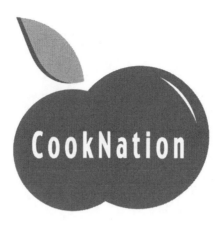

Other CookNation Titles

If you enjoyed 'The Skinny Takeaway Recipe Book' we'd really appreciate your feedback. Reviews help others decide if this is the right book for them so a moment of your time would be appreciated. Thank you.

You may also be interested in other '*skinny*' titles in the CookNation series.

You can find all the following great titles by searching under 'CookNation'.

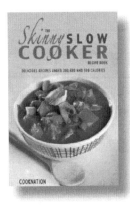

The Skinny Slow Cooker Recipe Book

Delicious Recipes Under 300, 400 And 500 Calories.

Paperback / eBook

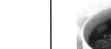
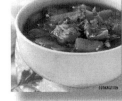

More Skinny Slow Cooker Recipes

75 More Delicious Recipes Under 300, 400 & 500 Calories.

Paperback / eBook

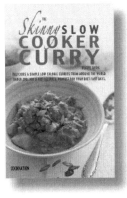

The Skinny Slow Cooker Curry Recipe Book

Low Calorie Curries From Around The World

Paperback / eBook

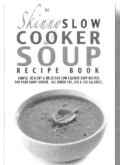

The Skinny Slow Cooker Soup Recipe Book

Simple, Healthy & Delicious Low Calorie Soup Recipes For Your Slow Cooker. All Under 100, 200 & 300 Calories.

Paperback / eBook

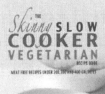
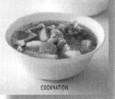
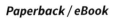

The Skinny Slow Cooker Vegetarian Recipe Book

40 Delicious Recipes Under 200, 300 And 400 Calories.

Paperback / eBook

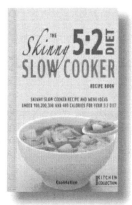

The Skinny 5:2 Slow Cooker Recipe Book

Skinny Slow Cooker Recipe And Menu Ideas Under 100, 200, 300 & 400 Calories For Your 5:2 Diet.

Paperback / eBook

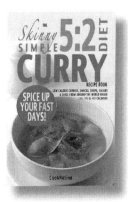

The Skinny 5:2 Curry Recipe Book

Spice Up Your Fast Days With Simple Low Calorie Curries, Snacks, Soups, Salads & Sides Under 200, 300 & 400 Calories

Paperback / eBook

The Skinny Halogen Oven Family Favourites Recipe Book

Healthy, Low Calorie Family Meal-Time Halogen Oven Recipes Under 300, 400 and 500 Calories

Paperback / eBook

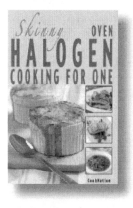

Skinny Halogen Oven Cooking For One

Single Serving, Healthy, Low Calorie Halogen Oven Recipes Under 200, 300 and 400 Calories

Paperback / eBook

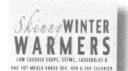
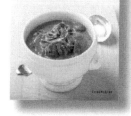

Skinny Winter Warmers Recipe Book

Soups, Stews, Casseroles & One Pot Meals Under 300, 400 & 500 Calories.

Paperback / eBook

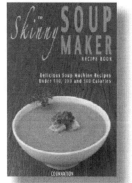

The Skinny Soup Maker Recipe Book

Delicious Low Calorie, Healthy and Simple Soup Recipes Under 100, 200 and 300 Calories. Perfect For Any Diet and Weight Loss Plan.

Paperback / eBook

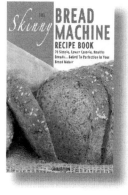

The Skinny Bread Machine Recipe Book

70 Simple, Lower Calorie, Healthy Breads...Baked To Perfection In Your Bread Maker.

Paperback / eBook

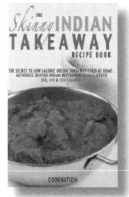

The Skinny Indian Takeaway Recipe Book

Authentic British Indian Restaurant Dishes Under 300, 400 And 500 Calories. The Secret To Low Calorie Indian Takeaway Food At Home

Paperback / eBook

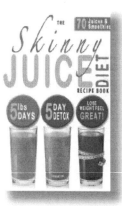

The Skinny Juice Diet Recipe Book

5lbs, 5 Days. The Ultimate Kick-Start Diet and Detox Plan to Lose Weight & Feel Great!

Paperback / eBook

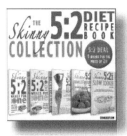

The Skinny 5:2 Diet Recipe Book Collection

All The 5:2 Fast Diet Recipes You'll Ever Need. All Under 100, 200, 300, 400 And 500 Calories

Available only on eBook

eBook

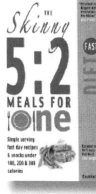

The Skinny 5:2 Fast Diet Meals For One

Single Serving Fast Day Recipes & Snacks Under 100, 200 & 300 Calories

Paperback / eBook

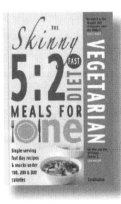

The Skinny 5:2 Fast Diet Vegetarian Meals For One

Single Serving Fast Day Recipes & Snacks Under 100, 200 & 300 Calories

Paperback / eBook

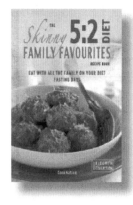

The Skinny 5:2 Fast Diet Family Favourites Recipe Book

Eat With All The Family On Your Diet Fasting Days

Paperback / eBook

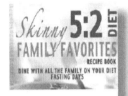

Available only on eBook

The Skinny 5:2 Fast Diet Family Favorites Recipe Book *U.S.A. EDITION*

Dine With All The Family On Your Diet Fasting Days

Paperback / eBook

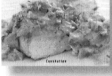

The Skinny 5:2 Diet Chicken Dishes Recipe Book

Delicious Low Calorie Chicken Dishes Under 300, 400 & 500 Calories

Paperback / eBook

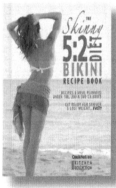

The Skinny 5:2 Bikini Diet Recipe Book

Recipes & Meal Planners Under 100, 200 & 300 Calories. Get Ready For Summer & Lose Weight...FAST!

Paperback / eBook

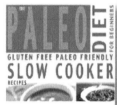

Available only on eBook

The Paleo Diet For Beginners Slow Cooker Recipe Book

Gluten Free, Everyday Essential Slow Cooker Paleo Recipes For Beginners

eBook

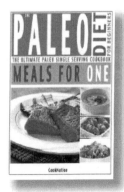

The Paleo Diet For Beginners Meals For One

The Ultimate Paleo Single Serving Cookbook

Paperback / eBook

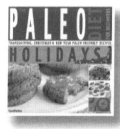

The Paleo Diet For Beginners Holidays

Thanksgiving, Christmas & New Year Paleo Friendly Recipes

Available only on eBook

eBook

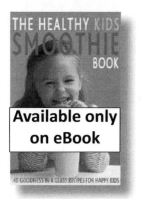

The Healthy Kids Smoothie Book

40 Delicious Goodness In A Glass Recipes for Happy Kids.

eBook

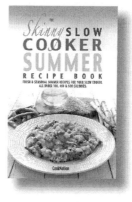

The Skinny Slow Cooker Summer Recipe Book

Fresh & Seasonal Summer Recipes For Your Slow Cooker. All Under 300, 400 And 500 Calories.

Paperback / eBook

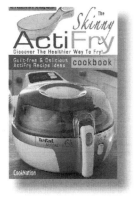

The Skinny ActiFry Cookbook

Guilt-free and Delicious ActiFry Recipe Ideas: Discover The Healthier Way to Fry!

Paperback / eBook

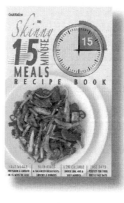

The Skinny 15 Minute Meals Recipe Book

Delicious, Nutritious & Super-Fast Meals in 15 Minutes Or Less. All Under 300, 400 & 500 Calories.

Paperback / eBook

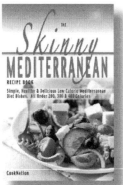

The Skinny Mediterranean Recipe Book

Simple, Healthy & Delicious Low Calorie Mediterranean Diet Dishes. All Under 200, 300 & 400 Calories.

Paperback / eBook

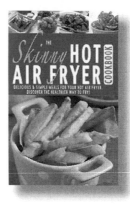

The Skinny Hot Air Fryer Cookbook

Delicious & Simple Meals For Your Hot Air Fryer: Discover The Healthier Way To Fry.

Paperback / eBook

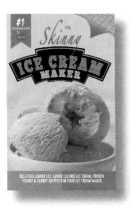

The Skinny Ice Cream Maker

Delicious Lower Fat, Lower Calorie Ice Cream, Frozen Yogurt & Sorbet Recipes For Your Ice Cream Maker

Paperback / eBook

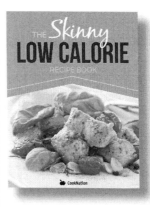

The Skinny Low Calorie Recipe Book

Great Tasting, Simple & Healthy Meals Under 300, 400 & 500 Calories. Perfect For Any Calorie Controlled Diet.

Paperback / eBook

Conversion Chart

Weights for dry ingredients:

Metric	Imperial
7g	¼ oz
15g	½ oz
20g	¾ oz
25g	1 oz
40g	1½oz
50g	2oz
60g	2½oz
75g	3oz
100g	3½oz
125g	4oz
140g	4½oz
150g	5oz
165g	5½oz
175g	6oz
200g	7oz
225g	8oz
250g	9oz
275g	10oz
300g	11oz
350g	12oz
375g	13oz
400g	14oz
425g	15oz
450g	1lb
500g	1lb 2oz
550g	1¼lb
600g	1lb 5oz
650g	1lb 7oz
675g	1½lb
700g	1lb 9oz
750g	1lb 11oz
800g	1¾lb
900g	2lb
1kg	2¼lb
1.1kg	2½lb
1.25kg	2¾lb
1.35kg	3lb
1.5kg	3lb 6oz
1.8kg	4lb
2kg	4½lb
2.25kg	5lb
2.5kg	5½lb
2.75kg	6lb

Conversion Chart

Liquid measures:

Metric	Imperial	Aus	US
25ml	1fl oz		
60ml	2fl oz	¼ cup	¼ cup
75ml	3fl oz		
100ml	3½fl oz	½ cup	½ cup
120ml	4fl oz		
150ml	5fl oz	¾ cup	¾ cup
175ml	6fl oz		
200ml	7fl oz	1 cup	1 cup
250ml	8fl oz	1¼ cups	
300ml	10fl oz/½ pt		
360ml	12fl oz		
400ml	14fl oz	2 cups	2 cups/1 pint
450ml	15fl oz	1 pint	2½ cups
600ml	1 pint		
750ml	1¼ pint	1¾ pints	1 quart
900ml	1½ pints		
1 litre	1½ pints		

Printed in Great Britain
by Amazon